How To Lose Weight Fast

Copyright 2006-2014 Robert E. Palma Jr.

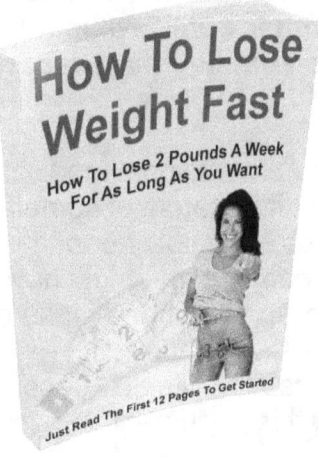

Disclaimer

This information is not presented by a medical practitioner and is for <u>inspirational purposes only</u>. The content is not intended to be a substitute for professional medical advice, diagnosis, or treatment. **Always seek the advice of your physician or other qualified health provider with any questions you may have regarding a medical condition**.

Never disregard professional medical advice or delay in seeking it because of something you have read. The author and publisher of this document and the accompanying materials have used their best efforts in preparing it and make no representation or warranties with respect to the accuracy, applicability, fitness, or completeness of the contents of this document.

The information contained in this document is strictly for inspirational purposes. Therefore, if you wish to apply ideas contained in this document, you are taking full responsibility for your actions. The author and publisher disclaim any warranties (express or implied), merchantability, or fitness for any particular purpose. The author and publisher shall in no event be held liable to any party for any direct, indirect, punitive, special, incidental or other consequential damages arising directly or indirectly from any use of this material, which is provided "as is", and without warranties.

As always, the advice of a competent legal, tax, accounting, medical or other professional should be sought. The author and publisher do not warrant the performance, effectiveness or applicability of any sites listed or linked to in this book. All links are for information purposes only and are not warranted for content, accuracy or any other implied or explicit purpose.

Table of Contents

Preface To This Book

The <u>purpose</u> <u>of</u> <u>this</u> <u>book</u> <u>is</u> <u>inspiration</u>. It is hoped that you will see that weight loss is not impossible, it is not difficult and it is not rocket science.

It is important to get specific advice for your needs from a medical, health professional. This book (itself) does not know you. So see your family doctor and health/fitness professional to find out what is good for you.

Don't delay. Get going now.

You don't need to read the whole book right now !

Just read Section 1, the Getting Started section. It is only 12 pages long! Find out how "doable" weight loss really is.

Section 1 Getting Started, Introduction

Congratulations! You've already taken an important step in losing weight! Chances are this isn't the first time you've looked into weight loss. You're not alone. Many people try and fail and try and fail repeatedly.

You need to understand that you cannot place all the blame on yourself. As a matter of fact, failure to lose weight or keep it off are usually due to the methods used, NOT a failure of the person attempting to lose weight.

The simple fact is that many fad diets and programs are difficult to follow because they aren't designed specifically for you. Instead, they are designed with a one-size-fits-all approach, which can be very frustrating for the individual.

We're all so very different when it comes to weight loss. Ultimately, the formula for weight loss is the same for all of us, but the way in which the formula is used effectively for each individual is what will make or break the diet plan.

And this is the key to success. By understanding weight loss, you can tailor a diet plan that works for you! There are five areas of weight loss that you need to understand so that this can be accomplished:

- Mindset
- The Magic Formula
- When to Eat and How Much
- What to Eat
- Exercise

Mindset

Food in our culture has been used as a focal point of celebration as well as a means to instant gratification.

What would Thanksgiving be like without the feast? Halloween without the candy? And do I really even need to mention the crazy eating that goes on through the biggest holiday season?

We've conditioned ourselves to regard food as a way to be happy. Not only that, but we use it for instant gratification. What happened when you scraped your knee as a child? Did you end up with a piece of candy to take the pain away?

We continue this pattern throughout our lives. We have bad days and indulge in a piece of cake or a bag of chips. A broken heart is often treated to something sinfully delicious. Of course, the food doesn't fix what's wrong.

The next time you are about to eat something that you know isn't a means to weight loss, think about why you are eating it. Are you hungry? If you are hungry, is there a better choice? If you aren't hungry, what else would make you feel better in the moment? Perhaps you could call a friend, go for a walk or listen to some uplifting music.

And when you do make a bad choice, don't beat yourself up. Acknowledge the mistake and move on. Make better choices for the rest of the day. Take it one day at a time and you'll find the challenge less daunting.

The Magic Formula

You've heard it before and you're going to hear it again. In order to lose weight you must eat less food and burn more calories.

Forget for the moment what to eat and what not to eat. We'll talk about that in a bit. For now, imagine that all you really have to do is remember not to eat more than you burn. Remember that in order to lose weight, you need to exercise every day to some extent so that you are burning more than you ate.

Calories in, minus, calories burned, should be a negative number to the tune of 500-1500 calories per day in order to lose 1-3 pounds per week. The average-sized person needs around 2000 calories per day just for the functions that the body must perform. This will vary plus or minus 300-500 calories depending on the person's height, age, sex, weight and activity level.

For simplicity's sake we are all going to pretend we are "average-sized" because if you follow this, you will lose weight. If you want to know your exact caloric needs, you can easily find that out with an online calorie calculator.

Based on the above information, your day should look something like this:

1500 calories eaten
500 calories burned

By doing this, you will have a 1000 calorie deficit every day (500 less eaten plus 500 burned).

When To Eat and How Much

Grazing is by far the best way to eat. By eating small amounts of food throughout the day, you are keeping your metabolism at an optimum level. Metabolism is the rate at which energy (measured in calories) is burned. When your metabolism is high, you burn calories more quickly. When your metabolism is low, your body stores more energy as fat.

When you starve yourself and skip meals, you're telling your body to keep metabolism low. Your body doesn't know when it's going to get energy again, so it stores most of what you eat as fat. When you graze throughout the day, you are constantly supplying your body with energy which tells the body that the energy is abundant and there's no need to store it as fat.

The key is to make sure that you are not taking in excessive amounts of energy. Excessive amounts of energy will also be stored as fat. What's needed here is an understanding of portion sizes.

Food labels are a great source of information on the amount of calories. Don't look at the percentages for now. Just look at the amount of calories per serving and how many servings are in the package.

Regarding the serving size, use measuring cups or spoons to measure out the food or eye-ball a portion based on the number of servings per package. A serving of meat is about the size of a deck of cards.

You're probably going to be shocked at first, but this is good. Now you know how you gained weight! A serving of ice cream, for example, is a half a cup. Take a half a cup of ice cream and put it in the bowl you would normally use for eating ice cream.

Think about the last time you ate potato chips and look at the amount of servings in the bag. One little old chocolate sandwich cookie has around 50 calories. How many do you usually eat?

It's hard, I know. We've all been there. How can one eat 15 potato chips and call it good? They are so small! But, if you want to lose weight you need to be aware of what you are putting in your mouth and you need to decide if that amount of calories is worth what you actually get to eat. Will it satisfy you?

By planning ahead and allowing yourself small servings of food throughout the day, you also lessen your risk of overeating at any one meal.

What To Eat

Now that you know how much and when, you need to know what to eat. You may not be able to adjust everything all at once, so ease yourself into making more healthful choices.

Carbohydrates will be around 50-60% of your daily intake. Your best choices here are vegetables, fruits, whole grains, nuts and seeds. Read labels carefully and stay clear of products made with refined flour. Often times, foods that seem like healthful choices such as crackers, breads and pastas are loaded with fat, sugar, preservatives and additives; none of which provide your body with any significant nutrients.

Protein choices should be lean. Great choices are chicken or turkey breast, fish and seafood, lean pork, lean beef and any plant source such as beans, legumes or soy. Poor choices are sausage, bacon (except for turkey bacon) and poor quality lunchmeat with fillers. Save the higher fat meats such as filet mignon for special occasions.

When it comes to fat, there's good fat and bad fat. Bad fat is saturated or trans fat and is found in high quantities in deep fried foods and the fattier meats in the previous paragraph. A lot of packaged refined products have a lot of saturated or trans fat as well.

Good fats are mono and polyunsaturated fats found in certain oils such as safflower, sunflower and olive oil as well as nuts, seeds and a few veggies or fruits such as avocado. You don't really need to worry about "adding" these to your diet. Replace bad fats with good fats instead.

Exercising

Last but certainly not least, exercise is the ultimate key to losing weight. You will not be able to lose weight and keep it off without adopting a lifestyle that includes physical activity. Also, when you lose weight, you want to lose fat, not muscle mass, so exercise!

Before beginning any strenuous exercise, you should have a physical and make sure you are up to the task. Your doctor may elect to start you out on more moderate forms of exercise such as yoga, Pilates or simply walking briskly.

By making at least 30 minutes of time per day to perform some sort of cardiovascular exercise, you will be well on your way to a healthier life and physique. This can be as simple as turning on the music and dancing your heart out or walking to work rather than driving. The idea is to work up a meaningful sweat at least once a day for 30-45 minutes.

Closing

In closing, remember to keep a positive attitude about your efforts. You've made a very important step by educating yourself on the basics of weight loss. Understanding these basics will help you make better choices and start down a road to weight loss success!

Section 2 Fast Tips For Weight Loss

Here are a series of tips for eating fewer calories and burning more calories throughout the day. These are instances that you frequently run into so if you read these through a few times then they will stick with you.

Losing Belly Fat Part 1

This series of articles focuses on approaches that do not require a gym, equipment or other hardware.

The good news is that losing belly fat is mostly the same procedure as losing fat on any part of the body. Different people have different areas of their body that seem to be the problem zone (for them). Differences can be due to their sex, due to genetics, and other reasons. In general, almost all people lose weight evenly across their whole body.

So you can follow a variety of routines to lose weight that will work for belly fat as well as other areas of the body.

The basic rule of losing weight (anywhere on the body) is to burn more calories in a day than you eat in a day. While some people try to use this approach on a weekly basis, a weekly approach is more likely to go awry. Try to do this on a daily basis: burn more than you eat.

There are many simple exercises (without any equipment) that you can do at home to build the ab muscles. There is a difference in opinion among experts as to whether building ab muscles actually makes you look better.

One viewpoint says that building muscles underneath a layer of fat will not make you look better. Seems to make sense – yes?

The other viewpoint says, lay on the ground and look at your stomach. It looks better now then when you are standing up – yes? Why is that? Well the fat is stretched out more and not being pulled over your belt line by gravity. So the theory here is that if you have stronger ab muscles, they will hold up your fat, at least a little more and you will or can, look better.

Well so much for the difference of opinions. One approach is to do both - lose fat, and build muscle. If you were only going to do one of them, which would you do? Ask yourself, what do you want. If the answer is to lose fat, then go ahead and lose fat. Make that your focus.

In future articles, exercise will be discussed that is specific to enhancing one's belly.

Losing Belly Fat Part 2

There are countless articles, even from this author that cover the basics of losing fat. They include:
- Reducing or completely cutting out junk food
- favoring whole foods
- watching and controlling fat content of what you eat
- watching and controlling calorie content of what you eat
- eating more small meals during the day rather than 3 big meals
- drinking water
- cutting down on alcohol

These are just some of the principles for what to eat.

The other side of the equation is exercise to burn fat. Here in this article we will focus on one exercise that is universal, easy to do, and does not require equipment.

Okay you probably guessed it – WALKING

Walking is an incredible exercise. It exercises muscles all over the body.

Walk briskly and swing your arms. You don't have to walk with a speed that causes you to get out of breath, but you are definitely not strolling.

How good is it?

Walking briskly, but not out of breath burns 6 to 9 calories per minute, depending upon your body weight.

30 minutes of walking is: 180 to 270 calories burned.

When losing weight you often want to burn approximately 500 calories a day. That means 500 calories more than you have been burning with your daily routine. So walking for 1 / 2 hour accomplishes half of your daily requirement.

So what does this have to do with your belly? Everything.

Walking burns calories, so it reduces fat. Walking builds muscle throughout the body, including your mid section. Walking is an important first step to reducing belly fat.
Always get the advice of your doctor or exercise professional before changing your daily routine or starting an exercise program.

Losing Belly Fat Part 3

In keeping with the approach of this series of articles, not to require any hardware, equipment or membership at a health club, here are 2 simple exercises that you can literally perform while sitting at your desk at the office.

Always get the advice of your doctor or exercise professional before changing your daily routine or starting an exercise program.

The previous articles spoke of:
- eating in a sensible way to reduce the number of calories you consume in a day
- burning calories through exercise
- building muscle over the whole body, through exercise

In this article the specific ab muscles and back muscles are addressed. Specifically, the upper, lower and oblique ab muscles and the muscles in the back, which support the ab muscles.

Exercise 1
When sitting at your desk, in a meeting, at the lunch table, anywhere – really, sit straight up. Straighten your back. Don't slump with your shoulders.

Your muscles are holding you body continuously. That's why when someone falls asleep in a meeting, their head bows down. The muscles are not holding it up.

So by sitting up straight you are working your ab and back muscles. You ARE exercising.

Pay attention to this. When you find you are slouching, sit back up immediately.

Exercise 2
Squeeze your ab muscles. This means, pull your belly button in. Then tilt your pelvis forward. If someone is watching you while you do this, it may appear that you are dancing while you are sitting.

You are not doing this continuously. Do a few reps of this, many times during the day.

Remember, if you want this to work, you have to do this every day. After a while it will be automatic.

Losing Weight In A Short Period Of Time Part 1

You need to lose weight every week to keep your motivation high. It could be easy to become discouraged if a week goes by and you seem to have the same weight. Here are important steps to achieve that.

Your mind set is important. Have a strong desire to lose weight successfully. With this in mind, you will be more determined to achieve it. This will help you not lose sight of your goal.

Be reasonable. Don't try to do the impossible like losing 30 pounds in a month or even 20 pounds in a month. This is probably not a good idea because it can have a big impact on the entire body bringing about other health problems.

Keep this simple. One pound lost per week is realistically the equivalent of around 3,500 calories, which is approximately losing 500 calories a day, through dieting and exercise.

Stay focused on the tasks that you need to do in order to lose weight rather than on how many pounds you wish to lose. By having the discipline to attend the exercise sessions that you have set for yourself, weight loss will occur as a result.

Write down your planned activities. Put it in a prominent place. Read it often. Always be honest with yourself.

Get the advice of your doctor or exercise professional. Exercise regularly. Plan the number of cardio exercise sessions that you need to for each week. Exercise at least 3 times per week if your professional advice recommends this, with every session lasting at least 30 minutes.

Eat a good diet. A balanced diet is very important if you want to lose weight quickly. Include fruits and vegetables in your meals to aid your digestion. Drink a lot of water to detoxify your body. Also, avoid junk food, and snacks.

Please avoid the junk food – candy, chips, peanut butter crackers, you know.

Keep the faith baby. You can do this.

Losing Weight In A Short Period Of Time Part 2

Do you eat dessert for breakfast? Most people do! Doughnuts, pastries, croissants, etc. In this article we will try to convince you not to do that. By the way, you would be surprised to find out that even plain croissants have quite a few calories, more than 100 calories.

Muffins (usually loaded with sugar) are just cake without icing. Popytarts are just slices of pie that you can cook in a toaster. Most commercial cereals are just loaded with sugar. None of these have many redeeming qualities. Stick to real food instead. Visit your local natural foods store and read the labels. Look for whole grain cereals without the added sugar. Read labels – take your glasses if you have reading glasses.

When you need a snack or a boost of energy, eat fresh fruit, or even dried fruit. Don't eat crackers, cookies, muffins, pizza, etc.

More carbohydrates = more calories. Consider the following choices:
Black beans, red beans, and lima beans pack almost 30 grams of carbohydrates into a serving. Green peas, snow peas, and sugar snap peas have only 10 grams of carbohydrates per serving.
Green beans have only 5 grams of carbohydrates.

These are huge differences. Make the smart choices.

Lettuce, spinach, chard, kale, cucumber, peppers, celery and other leafy greens offer some of the highest quality nutrition for a more natural low carbohydrate diet. Leafy green vegetables are high in phytonutrients and provide a good source of fiber.

Breads, pasta, and other starchy foods made with white flour have a great deal of carbohydrates. Visit your natural foods store and find whole grain breads. Many of these have little or no cholesterol and contain healthy ingredients like, flax, oat bran and whole wheat.

Don't worry about this. Don't think that it is too much to learn. Just apply it slowly over time. It will soon become second nature to you. Write some of these tips down on a 3 x 5 card and carry it in your pocket so it is always there when you are shopping. After a while you won't need it.

Losing Weight In A Short Period Of Time Part 3

Have you ever successfully lost weight only to regain it later? Most diets work, but it is also true to say that, ultimately, no diets work. Why is this so? Because when your diet is over, you're right back to your routine that got you overweight in the first place.

Here is an approach. Make small changes right now. The idea is to change your life-style, slowly, gradually. You will see weight loss quickly. It may not be a great deal of loss, but you will notice it. Over time the weight loss will be more and more.

By changing your life-style, this is a permanent change.

Don't think that this will be hard. It is not hard, and what you think is a big portion of the job to lose weight. Make up your mind to do this.

We are not making any drastic changes here – just gradual changes. Make one change each day. That's all.

In 10 days time you will have accomplished a great deal.

If you talk to people who've lost weight and kept it

off, they will likely tell you that they changed their lifestyle.

Here are just a few ideas of the gradual changes you can make.

1. No bag of chips to the couch. Change that. In fact, just stop eating on the couch entirely.
2. Eliminate the candy dishes around your house and on your desk at work. They are truly a menace to you. You'll save money too.
3. There are countless food products from soda pop, cookies, salad dressings, etc. that are loaded with sugar. Find sugar free substitutes.
4. Read the labels on the foods you buy in the grocery.
5. You don't have to put sugar in your tea. The Chinese don't !

You will start to see all the possibilities once you start these small gradual changes.

Keep the faith baby. You can do this.

Losing Weight In A Short Period Of Time Part 4

There are many practices for how to lose weight fast. Some of them, in fact more than half of them are quite simple. If you incorporate these into your daily life you will be pleasantly surprised at the results. Don't think of this as something hard to do. It is not hard – really. You can do this. Believe it.

The thoughts you have in your mind are a major part of what you are able to accomplish. You must believe that you can lose weight, and lose weight fast. Make it a happy pursuit. It is important that you be happy about this. Be confident that you can accomplish it.

Two things are happening. You are consuming calories and you are burning calories. As you become aware of how many calories are involved in both of these, you can lose weight.

It is important to exercise regularly. Get advice from your doctor or an exercise professional on how and how much to exercise. They will tell you what is just right for you. Exercise as much as you can, but be sure to be regular about it. Don't get carried away at first with a lot of exercise. If you try to do too much you could get frustrated and give up. Set a schedule and stick to it.

Cardio exercises like aerobics, jogging, swimming and brisk walking are good exercises to burn fat. As mentioned earlier, consult with a professional. You might be quite surprised at the effectiveness of brisk walking. Walking (briskly) has been said to be the best friend of someone who is losing weight – the best friend.

Remember the all-important principle that to lose weight, especially to lose weight fast, you must burn (with exercise) more calories than you consume (eat).

Keep at this. Make it fun. You can accomplish this. Always be patient, determined and persistent.

Losing Weight In A Short Period Of Time Part 5

There are many techniques for how to lose weight fast. Some of them are quite simple. If you practice enough of them in your daily life you will be pleasantly surprised at the results. This is not hard. You can do this.

What you are thinking, is a major part, of what you accomplish. You must believe that you can lose weight, and lose weight fast. Make it a happy pursuit. This is important. Be happy about it. Know that you can accomplish it.

In a lot of ways alcohol is not your "weight-loss friend". Even after a few sips of beer, your attitude to accomplishing weight loss could easily take a temporary back set. You could just forget about it for a while.

You must cut down on your alcohol intake. It is working against you in several ways. Alcohol slows down your metabolism rate and makes fat burning harder. This is just the opposite of what you want to do. You want your metabolism to be cranking along to burn calories – burn fat. With each beer you drink, you are taking in excessive calories that will also make you fatter. Therefore, if you want to slim down fast, the first thing that you need to do is to cut down, way down, on your alcohol intake. Drink lots of water to flush out the toxins and alcohol from your body so you can lose weight successfully.

Ever wondered why you get a headache from alcohol consumption? Drinking alcohol has been reported to form formaldehyde in your blood, hence you get a headache. Formaldehyde is not really a friendly chemical to have in your bloodstream.

Give fast food a vacation – a vacation from your life. Fast foods like burgers, French fries and cola are all filled with excessive calories. If you eat a lot of fast foods, you will tend to gain weight very easily. So if you want to know how to lose weight fast, stay away from fast food at all costs. Include vegetables and fruits in every meal that you eat. Healthy meals, make losing weight much easier.

Remember the foundational principle that to lose weight, you must burn (with exercise) more calories than you consume (eat).

Keep at this. You can do this. Be patient. Be determined. Your determination is your power to succeed. Be persistent.

Losing Weight In A Short Period Of Time Part 6

There are many, many techniques for losing weight. Learn enough of them and you will be on your way to slimming down. This is not hard. You can do this.

What you are thinking, is a major part, of what you accomplish. Believe that you can lose weight. Make it a happy pursuit. This is important. Be happy about it. Know that you can accomplish this.

Here we go:

Do not skip meals. You may want to skip meals but in order to lose weight your metabolism has to be kept high. In order for metabolism to be kept high there has to be fuel.

Drink green tea as an alternate for drinking coffee. It will stimulate your metabolism and it doesn't have the negative side effects like coffee.

Consume energy foods. They are a vital ingredient to increase your metabolism. Energy foods include whole grains, beans, vegetables and fruits.

Avoid High Fructose Corn Syrup. Read labels. This stuff is in a lot of prepared foods.

Surround yourself with supportive people and stay away from the negative people who find fault with you. Negative people are not helping you.

Get professional advice on exercising from your doctor or an exercise professional.

Set small goals at first. People are sometimes unable to achieve their fat loss goals because they focus on the ultimate end result. If your overall goal is to reduce your body fat by 10 percent, but focusing on that distant goal makes it seem to be too difficult, then you might feel tempted to quit your fat loss program altogether. So concentrate on what you're going to do to reduce it by one percent. Start slowly and you will find it much easier to stay positive.

Remember the foundational principle that you must burn (with exercise) more calories than you consume (eat).

Be patient. Be persistent.

Inspire yourself:
I AM doing this. Yes, I AM, I AM, I AM.

Losing Weight In A Short Period Of Time Part 7

By being aware of the principles of losing weight and the tips and tricks that really make a difference, you can see progress in how to lose weight fast, in a short period of time. You really can do this.

The most important aspect of how to lose weight fast, indeed at any rate, is your mind-set. You must really want to do it. You must be committed to following through to lose weight. Do not think that it will be difficult. Look in the mirror each morning and look into your own eyes and tell yourself, yes, this is what I want, and yes, this is that I will do.

The most fundamental principle of losing weight is to burn more calories than you eat.

Do not skip breakfast, it is a major mistake. Overnight your metabolic rate slows down. This slowing down will continue until you eat again. So eat breakfast to get the rate back up.

Drink water - lots of it. In between meals, when you are hungry, reach for water, not for a pop or anything with sugar. It is well known that often times, thirst is misinterpreted as hunger. Reach for water when you are hungry between meals.

Avoid sugar. Sugar facilitates the ability of the body to store fat. Nope, we don't want that.

No fried foods. You can grill or broil your meats and vegetables. Grilled and broiled foods are healthier than fried foods and easier to prepare. For vegetables, steaming is best.

Your eating should be like grazing. Eat less more often. Instead of the typical 3 meals a day, eat 5 to 6 smaller meals a day. This will keep you more full throughout the day, so you won't have urges for junk.

If you like spicy foods and they agree with you, then you will be happy to know that they increase metabolism.

Don't go to an all-you-can-eat restaurant. Just don't go there. It is definitely not part of how to lose weight fast.

No junk food. Completely cut it out of your diet. Completely. You can do this.

For desserts, choose fresh fruit.

Again, drink water - lots of it.

More Quick Tips Follow, 22 In All

1. Drink plenty of water. Our body needs a lot of water so give in to water. Water is not just way to flush out toxin but if you have more water in your body you will generally feel healthier and fitter. This will discourage any tendency to gorge. The best thing about water is that is has no calories at all.

2. Stay away from sweetened bottle drinks, especially sodas.

3. Include in your diet things that contain more water like watermelons, cantaloupe, etc. These things contain 90 to 95 % water so that there is nothing that you have to lose by enjoying them. They fill you up without adding pounds.

4. Eat fresh fruit instead of drinking fruit juice. Juice is often sweetened with sugar and corn syrup. When you eat fruit, you are taking in a lot of fiber, which is needed by the body, and fruits of course are an excellent source of vitamins.

5. Choose fresh fruit over processed fruits. Processed and canned fruits do not have as much fiber as fresh fruit and processed and canned fruits are nearly always sweetened.

6. Vegetables are your best bet when it comes to losing pounds. Nature has a terrific spread when it comes to choosing vegetables. Leafy green vegetables are your best bet. Try to include a small salad in you diet.

7. Watch what you eat. Keep a watchful eye on every thing that goes in. Sometimes the garnishes can richer than the food itself.

8. Control your sweet tooth. Remember that sweet things generally mean more calories. It is natural that we have cravings for sweet things especially chocolates and other confectionary. Go easy on theses things and each time you consume something sweet understand that it is going to add on pounds somewhere.

9. Eat only when you are hungry. Some of us have the tendency to eat whenever we see food. We use parties as an excuse to stuff our selves. Understand that the effect of a whole week of dieting can be wasted by just one day's party food. Whenever you are offered something to eat that you don't really need or want, you do not have to decline it completely, but just break of a nibble so that you appear to mind your manners and at the same time can watch your diet.

10. Quit snacking in between meals. This is especially true for those who have to travel a lot. They feel that the only time they can get a

bite to eat is snacks and junk food. The main problem with most snacks and junk food is that they are usually less filling and contain a lot of fat and calories. Just think about French fries…tempting but terribly fattening.

11. Snack on vegetables if you must. You might get the pangs of hunger in between meals. It is something that you can very well control. Or even better, try munching on celery or carrots. They are an excellent way to satisfy those hungry pangs and carrots are good for your eyes and teeth. True, you might end up being called Bugs Bunny, but its miles better to be called Bugs Bunny than fatso.

12. Go easy on tea and coffee. Tea and coffee do not cause weight gain by themselves. It's when you add the cream and sugar that they become fattening. Did you know that having a cup of tea or coffee that has cream and at least two cubes of sugar is as many calories as having a piece of rich chocolate cake?

13. Stay away from fried foods. The more fried foods that you avoid, the less weight you will gain. Even if the external oil is drained away, there is still a lot of hidden oil in it so stay away from fried foods.

14. Instead of frying food try baking them without fat. Baking is by far a healthier method of preparing food than frying.

15. Do not skip meals. It slows your metabolism down. Especially do not skip breakfast. You need to have at 4, 5, or 6 smaller meals every day.

16. Make chocolates an occasional luxury and not a routine. Even the so-called dark chocolates are not good for you because there is still a good amount of sugar in the recipe and they also have cream in them.

17. High Fiber multigrain breads are better than white breads. They are not only better in terms of the fiber content but also in terms of the protein content.

18. Steam your vegetables instead of boiling them. This is probably the healthiest way to eat cabbages, cauliflowers and a host of other vegetables.

19. Avoid crash diets. They can be bad for health and you will gain what you have lost once you take a break from the diet. Crash diets are not a solution to weight loss. Changing your life-style is a solution. Take a look at it in this way. Do you think that it is possible for a person to survive on a crash diet for the rest of his or her life? Certainly not! So at some time or the other, you will have to give up the crash diet and then you will see for yourself that a crash diet does more harm than good on the long run.

20. Develop a habit of chewing all food including liquid food and soft foods like milk, sweets, ice creams at least 10 to 20 times. Chewing (mastication) and saliva in your mouth are an essential part of digestion.

21. When you do notice a change (reduction) in your weight, then reward yourself. But not with food. Go for a movie or buy yourself something like a new dress or a trinket. This is something that can keep you going. It is a good idea to save on the money that you wanted to spend on ice creams and chocolates and then treat your self to something more substantial.

22. Turn on music and dance. Let your hair down. Close the door of your room, turn on your sound system to the highest volume possible (without torque-off your neighbors) and then do the wildest dance that you can think of. Pretend that you are Michael Jackson or Madonna (you will never see them keeping still) and do ever boogie-woogie move that you know.

Section 3 Calories Found In Food

These are approximate only, but will give you an idea of some foods to favor and others to stay away from in your daily routine.

Apples:
- o 1 slice apple pie: 400 calories
- o 1 cup sweetened apple sauce: 190 calories
- o 1 cup unsweetened applesauce: 100 calories
- o 1 sliced raw apple, 1 cup: 60 calories

Avocado
- o Qty. 1 is: 400 calories

Banana
- o Qty. 1 is 100 calories

Beef and vegetable stew
- o 1 cup is: 230 calories

Beef Gravy
- o 1 cup is: 140 calories

Beer

- 12 Oz regular: 160 calories
- 12 Oz Light: 110 calories

Blue cheese salad dressing
- 1 tablespoon: 80 calories
- 4 tablespoon: 320 calories

Broccoli
- 1 cup cooked: 40 calories

Butter
- 1 pat: 38 calories
- 1 tablespoon: 110 calories
- 1 cup: 800 calories

Cake, Spice, with icing
- 1 slice: 400 calories

Cashews Dry Roasted
- 1 oz: 180 calories
- 1 cup: 800 calories

Celery
- 1 stalk: 4 calories

Cherry Pie
- 1 slice: 425 calories

Chocolate Chip Cookie

- 1 cookie: 50 calories

Coconut Raw Shredded
- 1 cup: 300 calories

Cola Pop Drink
- Regular 12 oz: 180 calories
- Diet 12 oz: 0 calories

Corn Chips
- 1 oz: 150 calories

Corn Flakes
- 1 oz: 110 calories

Corn Cooked
- 1 cup from frozen: 140 calories
- From 1 ear: 60 calories

Cottage Cheese 2% Lo Fat
- 1 cup: 200 calories

Cream Cheese
- 1 oz: 100 calories

Cream pie
- 1 slice: 480 calories

Danish Fruit Pastry

- 1 piece: 240 calories

Date
- 1 each: 25 calories

Doughnut plain
- 1 each: 215 calories

Egg, fried
- 1 each: 95 calories

English Muffin
- 1 each: 140 calories

Fish Sandwich
- 1 each: 490 calories

Fish Stick
- 1 each: 75 calories

French Dressing
- 1 tablespoon: 90 calories
- 4 tablespoons 360 calories

Ginger ale
- 12 oz: 125 calories

Graham crackers
- 1 each: 35 calories

Grape Nuts cereal
- o 1 oz: 100 calories

Half and Half
- o 1 tablespoon: 25 calories

Hamburger Sandwich
- o Small patty: 250 calories
- o Large patty: 450 calories

Ice Cream, Vanilla
- o Regular 1 cup: 280 calories
- o Rich 1 cup: 350 calories
- o Soft Serve 1 cup: 380 calories

Imitation Creamer
- o 1 tablespoon: 25 calories

Jelly
- o 1 tablespoon: 50 calories

Jelly Beans
- o 1 oz: 110 calories

Lemon Lime Soda Pop
- o 12 oz: 150 calories

Lettuce Raw

- 1 leaf: 1 calories

Lima Beans cooked:
- 1 cup: 260 calories

Macaroni, cooked
- 1 cup: 190 calories

Margarine
- 1 tablespoon: 50 to 120 calories (read the label)

Milk Chocolate
- 1 oz: 155 calories

Mixed Nuts
- 1 oz: 180 calories

Oatmeal raisin cookies
- 1 each: 70 calories

Olive Oil
- 1 tablespoon: 130 calories

Orange soda pop
- 12 oz: 180 calories

Orange, raw
- 1 each: 60 calories

Peach pie
- o 1 slice: 410 calories

Pears
- o 1 each 80-120 calories depending upon type

Pecan Pie
- o 1 slice: 585 calories

Pop corn, air popped, no oil
- o 1 cup: 35 calories

Potato, Baked
- o No skin: 150 calories
- o With skin: 220 calories

Potato, French Fired
- o Just 1 strip: 18 calories

Pound cake
- o 1 slice: 120 calories

Pretzel sticks
- o 1 stick: 1 calories

Pudding, Chocolate
- o 1 / 2 cup: 160 calories

Pudding, Rice
- o 1 / 2 cup: 160 calories

Raisin Bread
- o 1 slice: 70 calories

Rice, white cooked
- o 1 cup: 230 calories

Saltines
- o 1 cracker: 15 calories

Shredded wheat cereal, no frosting
- o 1 oz: 100 calories

Sour cream
- o 1 tablespoon: 25 calories

Spinach cooked
- o 1 cup: 55 calories

Sugar, white
- o 1 packet: 30 calories

Swiss cheese
- o 1 oz: 110 calories

Tea, unsweetened

- 1 cup: 0 calories

Tomato juice
- 1 cup: 40 calories

Vegetables, mixed
- 1 cup: 75 calories

Waffle
- 1 slice: 220 calories

Wheat bread
- 1 slice: 65 calories

Whipping cream
- 1 tablespoon: 65 calories

Wine, table
- 3.5 oz: 85 calories

Yogurt Low fat
- 8 oz: 150 calories

Zucchini
- 1 cup: 35 calories

Section 4 Magic Foods, Negative Calorie Foods

The only true low calorie food is water. It has zero calories. When you eat, you digest, and that process of digesting takes energy. There are foods that have been said to consume more calories (in the digesting process) than the amount of calories in the food itself.

The idea here is that eating these foods are unlikely to add any weight to you. Sometimes they are called Magic Foods (from the weight loss standpoint) or Negative Calorie Foods.

How this works in _your_ body is something that you can discuss with your doctor and professional weight trainer.

Vegetables

- Asparagus
- Broccoli
- Cabbage
- Carrot
- Cauliflower
- Celery
- Cucumber

- Endive
- Green Beans
- Lettuce
- Onion Papaya
- Radishes
- Spinach
- Turnip
- Zucchini

Now let's look at the fruits.

Fruits

- Apple
- Cranberries
- Grapefruit
- Lemon
- Mango
- Orange
- Pineapple
- Raspberries
- Strawberries
- Tangerine

Section 5 Burning Calories Examples

This section will give you an idea how what it takes to burn calories with a few common activities. This is a short section of the book but it is a good one to read over a few times so that you remember it.

You might have a few times during the day when you have some free time and you could use it to burn some calories or you could simply sit in one spot. The following information will open your eyes as to the difference.

Another idea is that when you park your car in the mall parking lot, you could pick the closest spot to the entrance, or you could pick the farthest away. The following information will help you decide.

In the following information, a range of calories burned is given. The more you weigh the more you burn with these activities.

There are some real eye-openers in the list. For example, compare climbing stairs with aerobic training and basketball. Do you have opportunities to "take the stairs" rather than the elevator?

As always, check with your doctor and professional trainer before changing your life-style or putting yourself on an exercise routine.

These numbers are:
Calories burned in 1 minute

- Aerobic training: 7 to 11 calories
- Basketball: 7 to 11 calories
- Bowling: 1 to 2 calories
- Climbing Stairs: 9 to 11 calories
- Cycling at 10 MPH: 5 to 8 calories
- Golf (pull your cart): 4 to 7 calories
- Golf (ride power cart): 2 to 3 calories
- Hiking: 4 to 7 calories
- Jogging: 9 to 14 calories
- Running: 11 to 17 calories
- Sitting: 1 to 1.8 calories
- Skating: 5 to 9 calories

- Cross Country Skiing: 9 to 11 calories
- Swimming (crawl at medium pace): 7 to 11 calories
- Walking (briskly but not out of breath): 6 to 9 calories
- Tennis: 6 to 10 calories
- Weight training: 6 to 9 calories